D1081425

THE COUCH POTATO'S

GUIDE TO GETTING FIT

THE COUCH POTATO'S GUIDE TO GETTING FIT

Copyright © Summersdale Publishers Ltd, 2019

Text by Sophie Martin
Illustrations by Hamish Braid
Character design by Kate Cooper

All rights reserved.

No part of this book may be reproduced by any means, nor transmitted, nor translated into a machine language, without the written permission of the publishers.

Condition of Sale
This book is sold subject to the condition that it shall not, by way of trade or otherwise, be lent, resold, hired out or otherwise circulated in any form of binding or cover other than that in which it is published and without a similar condition including this condition being imposed on the subsequent purchaser.

An Hachette UK Company
www.hachette.co.uk

Summersdale Publishers Ltd
Part of Octopus Publishing Group Limited
Carmelite House
50 Victoria Embankment
LONDON
EC4Y 0DZ
UK

www.summersdale.com

Printed and bound in the Czech Republic

ISBN: 978-1-78685-732-3

Substantial discounts on bulk quantities of Summersdale books are available to corporations, professional associations and other organizations. For details contact general enquiries: telephone: +44 (0) 1243 771107 or email: enquiries@summersdale.com.

THE COUCH POTATO'S

GUIDE TO GETTING FIT

summersdale

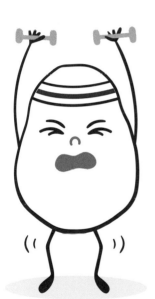

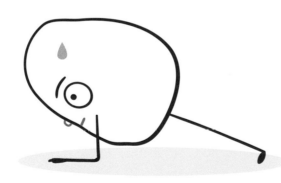

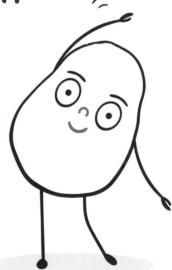

SIMPLE EXERCISES TO GET IN SHAPE

Jamie Easton

Neither the author nor the publisher can be held responsible for any loss or claim arising out of the use, or misuse, of the suggestions made herein. Consult your doctor before undertaking any new forms of exercise.

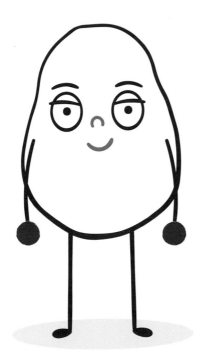

CONTENTS

INTRODUCTION

Welcome to *The Couch Potato's Guide to Getting Fit!*
My name is Instructor Pot and I'll be guiding you through all sorts of exercises to get you off the couch and into your teeny tiny spandex. (That's a joke – I would never force anyone to wear ill-fitting, uncomfortable sportswear unless they truly wanted to.)

This book begins with easy stretches, perfect for anyone who will feel out of their depth even saying the word "exercise". They focus on all parts of the body to improve flexibility and balance and will help make the subsequent exercises easier to perform.

The next section will look at some very simple exercises that you can perform from the comfort of your own home. They are primarily focused on toning and strengthening your muscles. If this is your first time partaking in any physical activity for a while, choose a couple of stretches followed by just one or two exercises. Continue with these until you feel confident, then gradually increase the amount you do. Try to pick exercises that focus on different parts of the body so you don't put too much stress on one area. However, if you suffer from a particular injury or niggle in a certain part of your body, avoid doing any exercises that focus on it or perform them very gently.

Once you've spent a while mastering your strengthening exercises, it's time to tackle the aerobic exercises. These vary from gentle – where you'll only feel your heartbeat quicken slightly – to fairly difficult – where you might start to perspire and you'll notice your breathing change. Aerobic exercises are a great option for steady weight loss if you perform them frequently, and the longer the sessions you do the more calories you'll burn. As with any exercise, start slowly and make your sessions short, then gradually build up your speed and the length of time you perform them for.

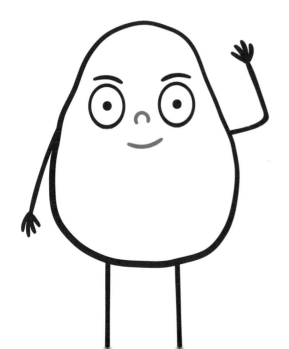

If you are enjoying your daily exercises and you have noticed a difference in the way you look and feel, but you want to challenge yourself even more, then the last section is for you. These exercises are quite a lot harder than any others in the book, so don't worry if you don't think you are ready for them quite yet. Give it another few months and the exercise world will be your oyster. To help you to build up to these harder routines, to perfect your posture and technique, and to give you confidence, there are exercises in the earlier sections that will set you up for the big ones.

That's all from me for now, so I will (hopefully) see you shortly when you turn the page to a new chapter of your healthier and happier life.

BEFORE YOU BEGIN

If you want to start feeling fitter and healthier, exercise is the best way to begin as long as you're making an effort to change other areas of your lifestyle too. Before you begin your exercise adventure, take heed of and put into practice the following tips and advice:

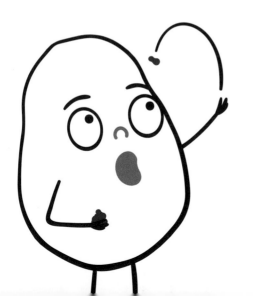

Eat better – try to have three balanced, wholesome meals a day. You want to eat foods that release energy slowly, e.g. starchy carbs (bread, rice, pasta and potatoes – argh!). A common diet issue amongst many of us is iron deficiency, so make sure you eat your greens – breakfast cereals are also a good source of iron. Another big misconception is that you'll lose weight if you skip breakfast. In fact, the opposite is true. To keep you going until lunchtime, try having porridge, high-fibre cereals, wholemeal toast or poached/boiled eggs.

Snack less – as well as snacking less, you should choose what you snack on more carefully. Chocolate bars, crisps, and the like are high in sugar but low in energy. However, if you opt for snacks such as nuts, seeds, raisins and fruit, you'll notice a difference in how much longer you'll feel full for. There's no harm in snacking in between breakfast and lunch and lunch and dinner, especially when exercising, just as long as they are the healthy type of snacks.

Hydrate more – one big advantage of staying hydrated is that you'll feel fuller. You may have heard that if you drink a glass of water before any meal you will eat what your body needs, not what you think it needs. The recommended daily water intake is 6–8 glasses for an adult.

It's also a good idea to cut down on fizzy drinks and alcohol, as they contain empty calories (calories that don't give you proper energy).

Seek medical attention – if you are worried about your physical condition or are on medication, seek advice from your doctor before doing any of the exercises in this book.

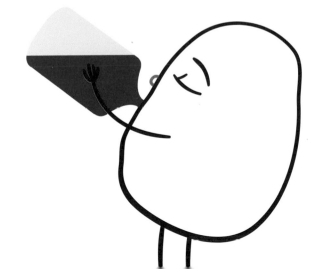

BENEFITS OF EXERCISE

There are countless reasons why you should exercise more, including:

Sleeping better – it is recommended that we have 6–8 hours' sleep per night. However, the reality is that most of us are having a lot less. Most of the time this is caused by stress, anxiety and a surplus of energy. Exercise burns energy, thus it will make us feel more tired in the evening. Our lifestyles have become a lot more sedentary compared with our ancestors' and it's unnatural for our bodies to be sitting down all day. Complement the exercises in this book with walking up the stairs instead of taking the elevator and taking a stroll to the local convenience store instead of driving. If you continue exercising, you'll notice the difference in your sleeping patterns and will feel fresher and revitalized.

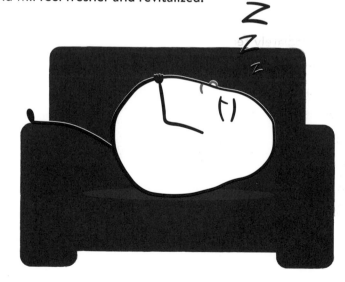

Less anxiety – exercise releases feel-good endorphins that help to relieve stress and anxiety and improve your mood. Many people go to yoga classes just for the reason that it relaxes them – the exercise, strengthening and better flexibility are just added bonuses for some.

More confident – as you start to lose weight, see muscles you never thought you had and feel fitter, you'll immediately feel better about yourself and have higher self-esteem. Additionally, as you sleep more and feel less anxious and stressed as a result of exercising, this will in turn make you feel more confident – you will change in many ways as an individual, but all these changes are positive and you won't regret them. The main thing is that you *maintain* the adjustments in your life for a happier, longer existence!

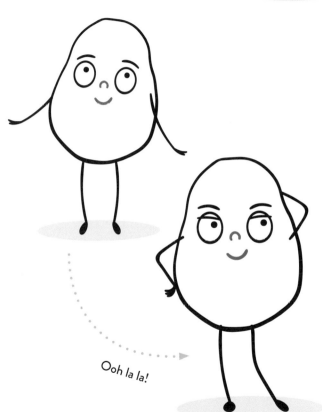

Ooh la la!

EQUIPMENT

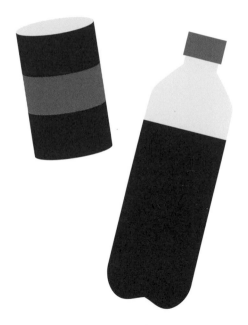

This book is for exercise beginners so we don't expect you to have a treadmill and bench press handily situated in your living room. However, you will need a couple of items from your kitchen cupboards for some of the exercises. If you are sticking to a regular exercise routine, and have been for a while, we've also included some simple, effective and cheap equipment that will take your sessions to the next level.

Tinned food – whether the food they contain is fresh or it expired months ago, these cans are the perfect size to hold in your hands and the perfect weight. (Don't cheat by using empty tins – there's no sense of achievement in that!)

Water bottles – another household item that is easy to hold and a good weight. You can even take a sip from them while resting. If you want to use them as heavier makeshift weights, replace the water with sand.

Resistance bands – these are super-cheap, available online and in sports shops, and are a great investment if you plan to do regular exercises. They are made from latex – which means they are stretchy but resistant at the same time – and come in varying sizes. They are used regularly for exercises that focus on arm and leg strengthening. For example, a very basic arm exercise would be to take the band in both hands and hold it out in front of you so your arms are shoulder-width apart. Then stretch the band as far as you can. After a while, you will be able to feel your shoulder and back muscles working. A basic leg exercise using the band is to tie the band around your ankles,

then stand on one leg and push the other leg out sideways away from the standing leg. The resistance you feel will strengthen your inner and outer thigh muscles.

Wrist and ankle weights – these are more expensive than resistance bands, but they are more convenient as you just strap them to your ankles or wrists and perform the exercises as you would normally.

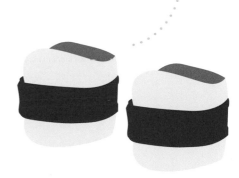

SIMPLE STRETCHES

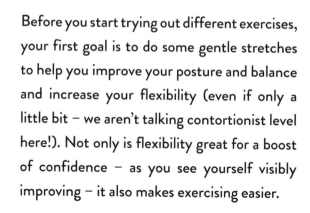

Before you start trying out different exercises, your first goal is to do some gentle stretches to help you improve your posture and balance and increase your flexibility (even if only a little bit – we aren't talking contortionist level here!). Not only is flexibility great for a boost of confidence – as you see yourself visibly improving – it also makes exercising easier.

SEATED CHEST LIFT

Midway through this movement, it may look like you're gesturing for a hug, so try not to do it in public – unless you enjoy intimate moments with strangers. Once you complete a set, you'll notice that your chest feels a lot more open. After performing this stretch frequently you'll notice a difference in your posture too.

Stretches: chest, shoulders and back

Sit on a stable chair

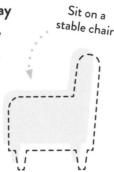

1 Sit on a sturdy chair with no wheels or arms, or sit in the middle of your couch if you don't have the correct chair (although this isn't the best option as the cushions will make you feel like you're sinking, not extending).

2 Make sure your feet are flat on the floor and your back is not leaning but straight.

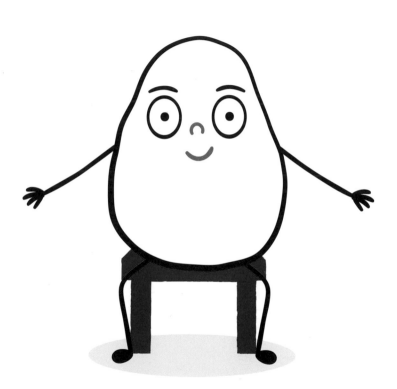

3 Extend your arms out in a low "V" shape, your hands pointing towards the ground, keeping your shoulders and neck relaxed (you will feel like you are pulling your shoulders down your back).

4 Gently push your chest forwards and up – this will naturally make your arms move back slightly. If you want a bigger stretch, gently force your arms back a little more.

5 Hold for 10 seconds and then have a rest. Find your original position, with your feet flat on the floor and your back straight and unsupported, then repeat another 4 times (5 in total).

SEATED UPPER-BODY TWIST

If done regularly, this exercise will help you strengthen your upper back and give it more flexibility. Arms crossed, you will feel like you're protecting yourself from the exercise before you even start, but relax and you'll soon start to enjoy it.

Stretches: upper back

Sit on a stable chair

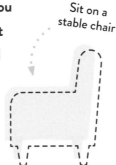

1 Sit on a sturdy chair with no wheels or arms. A couch will do if you don't have an alternative. Make sure your feet are flat on the floor and your back is not leaning but dead straight.

2 Bend your elbows and cross your arms so that both hands are resting on the opposite shoulders.

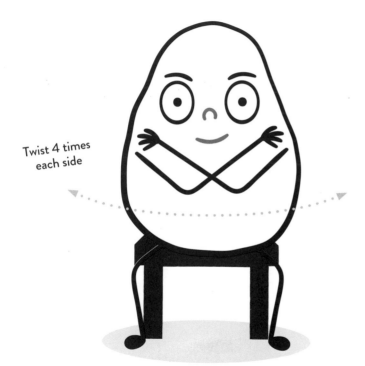

Twist 4 times
each side

3 Twist your upper back to the right as far as you can and move your head so it faces the same direction. Hold this position for 5 seconds. Try not to tense your thighs as you twist and keep your hips facing forwards. This will make the stretch more effective.

4 Return to facing forwards and repeat on the other side.

5 Repeat 4 more times on each side.

SEATED KNEE LIFT

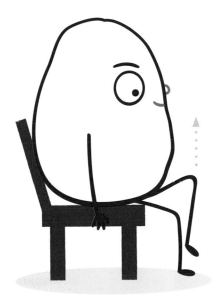

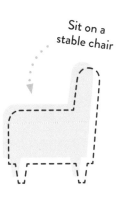

Sit on a stable chair

Feel like you are Bruce Lee ready for a brawl (albeit a seated one).

Stretches: hip rotators

1 Dig out that trusty chair again (the one with no wheels or arms) and sit on it with your feet flat on the floor and your back straight and unsupported.

2 Grab the sides of the chair with your hands for support.

3 Bend your right leg and lift it as far as feels comfortable, then lower it with control.

4 Repeat with the left leg and again until you have completed the lift 5 times with each leg.

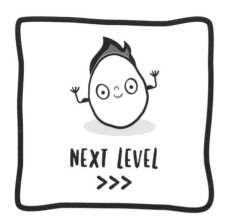

NEXT LEVEL
>>>

To give your hamstrings a stretch too, perform the seated knee lift but after lifting your leg, try straightening it out until you can feel a nice pull at the back of your leg. Then bend your knee back to the position of the seated knee lift and then gently lower your leg to the floor.

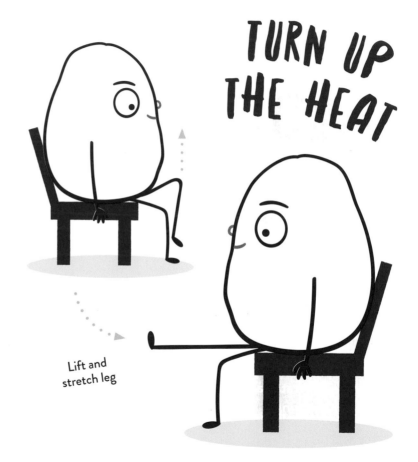

TURN UP THE HEAT

Lift and stretch leg

GOOD TOES, NAUGHTY TOES

As they are the part of your body furthest from your head, your feet are often forgotten about (poor soles!). Get them moving again with this exercise to improve blood circulation and ankle flexibility.

Stretches: metatarsals, ankles, hamstrings

Sit on a stable chair

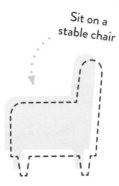

1 Go back to your chair (or just remain seated) with your feet flat on the floor. You can lean your back against the support of the chair for this exercise but, if you want, you can hold the sides of the chair for some extra support.

2 Raise your straight right leg off the ground in front of you and start by flexing your ankle so your toes are pointing

up at the sky. Hold for a few seconds – you should feel a pull on your hamstrings – and then point the foot so your ankle is elongated.

3   In the process of flexing and pointing your feet, try to think about going through your foot one part at a time so that you are using and strengthening all your muscles in that region.

4   Hold your leg with a pointed foot for a few seconds and then repeat the movement another 4 times with the same foot.

5   Lower the right leg and repeat on the other side.

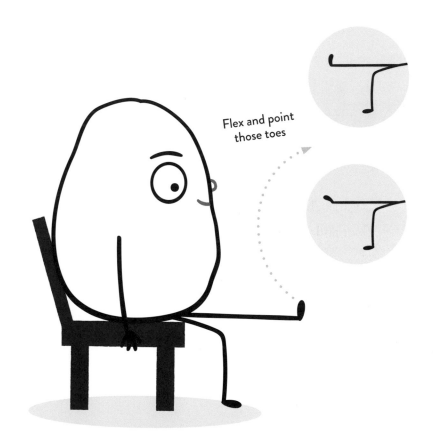

Flex and point those toes

SEATED HEAD TILT

Even though it's an exercise, this feels so good that you'll want to do it again and again. (Always trust the words of a potato.)

Stretches: neck

Sit on a stable chair

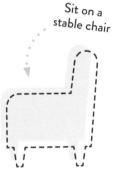

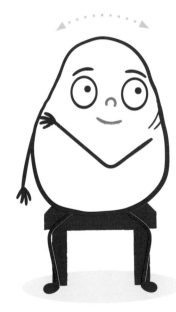

1 Sit on a chair with your feet flat on the floor and your back leaning flat against the support.

2 Bend your elbow and place your hand on top of the opposite shoulder and press down on it.

3 Tilt your head the opposite way to the side where your hand is pressing down on your shoulder.

4 Hold this stretch for 5 seconds and repeat on the other side.

5 Repeat another 2 times on each side.

CHILD POSE (RESTING POSE)

This pose is popular in yoga and is one of my favourites, as it means that it's time to take a short rest. It is frequently recommended throughout the book as a pose to rest in after completing an exercise.

Stretches: arms, shoulders and back

1 Kneel on the floor with your backside lifted off the ground.

2 Position your feet so they are almost touching and your knees are pointing outwards.

3 Move your butt back with the aim of sitting on your heels. The majority of us can't do this, so don't worry if your backside is hovering in mid-air. Your head should be touching or almost touching the ground and your arms should be stretched out, palms down, in front of you. You can also place your arms by your sides if this feels easier for you. You are resting after all, so you want to feel as relaxed as possible.

GLUTE FLEX

This stretch will cause an "ouch" and "ah" moment simultaneously.

Stretches: glutes

1 Lying on your back, bend both knees so that your feet are flat on the floor.

2 Lift your right leg and rotate it so that your right ankle is sitting in front of your left knee.

3 Grab the back of your left thigh – you may need to sit up a little to do this – and pull it towards your body as far as it will go. If you did change your position to grab your leg, make sure you return to lying down for the stretch. You should feel a pull running through your right glute.

4 Hold the position for 5 seconds or whenever is enough for you, then return to the original position with your feet flat on the floor.

5   Repeat on the other side and then another 2 times on each leg.

6   If you aren't able to lift both legs off the floor, just do the exercise up to step 2 and repeat on the other side.

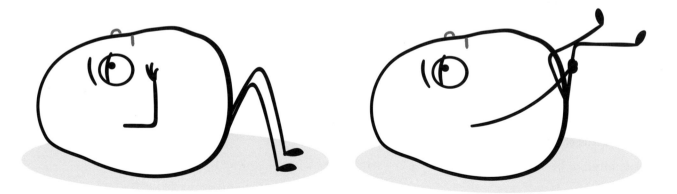

KNEELING LUNGE

This is a great exercise to open up the hips. Next stop: splits... (or a banana split!).

Stretches: hip flexors

1 Position yourself with your left knee and your right foot flat on the floor with your right knee at a right angle, and place your body weight in the middle of the two. You can do this stretch with your left foot either pointed or bent so the ball of the foot is supporting you.

2 Make any adjustments to your right foot if necessary so you have enough room to lunge. Place your hands on your right thigh.

3 To start the lunge, bend your right knee some more and lower your body further to the ground, keeping your back straight. Concentrate on making your body weight heavy – this will make the stretch more effective – and ensure your hips are facing forward.

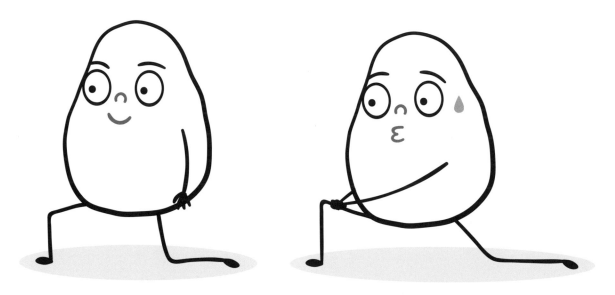

4 Stay in this position for 10 seconds and then come up.

5 Repeat on the other side.

Important: your front knee shouldn't go over your toes when you lunge. If it does, adjust your position so that your legs are further apart.

BACK STRETCH

This exercise feels wonderful but take it slowly because if you haven't been physically active for a while your back will be very stiff!

Stretches: lower back

1 Lie face down with your elbows bent and your lower arms and hands on the floor – hands should be palms down, just below your shoulders.

2 Push down with your hands into the ground, and lift your head and upper back off the floor slightly. Feel how your lower back muscles are activating.

3 Hold for 5 seconds then lower yourself back down to the floor.

4 Repeat this 4 more times with rests in between.

Extend your arms and push your head up for a good back stretch

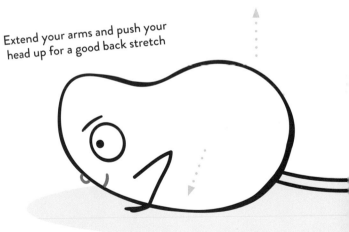

STANDING SIDEWAYS BEND

You may think I'm trying to pull your leg, but this exercise will also give you a satisfying stretch. Don't say I didn't tell you so.

Stretches: sides of the body

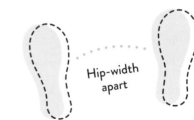

Hip-width apart

1 Sorry, you're going to have to stand for this exercise.
Good thing is you'll be almost stationary the entire time.
Place your feet hip-width apart, your arms by your sides and
make sure your weight isn't back on your heels.

2   Slide your right hand down the outside of your right leg and allow your left shoulder to raise. This should create a stretch along the left side of your body. Concentrate on your hips facing forward and your left shoulder pointing straight up to the sky. This will give you the best stretch.

3   Hold this side stretch for 5 seconds and then return to your normal standing position.

4   Slide down on the other side and then repeat 4 more times each way.

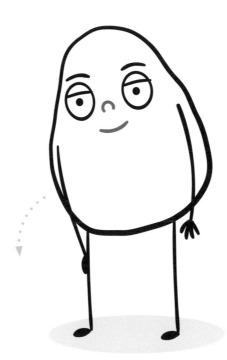

CALF STRETCH

Oooo, your legs will love you for this. You may need to give them a bit of an oil first if you haven't used them in a while!

Stretches: calf muscles

1 Stand facing a wall and position the tips of your toes on your right foot so they touch the bottom of the wall.

2 Resting your hands against the wall for support, step back with your left leg and place your foot flat on the ground. It should be at least one stride away from your right foot.

3 Now bend your right knee. Your left leg should be straight with the heel firmly on the floor for achieving the most effective stretch.

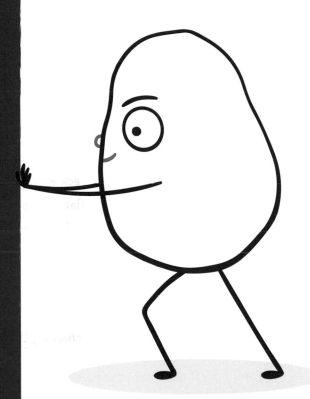

4   Hold this position for 10 seconds and then swap sides.

5   If you can't feel much of a stretch, move your back foot further away from your front foot.

6   Perform the stretch another 4 times on each side.

STANDING HAMSTRING STRETCH

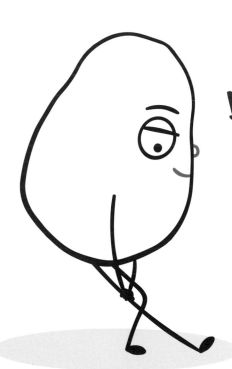

While the calf stretch on the previous page focuses on the lower leg muscles, this stretch is to improve your hamstring flexibility.

Stretches: hamstrings

1 Standing upright, extend your right leg in front of you with the heel touching the floor. Rest your hands gently on your right thigh.

2 Keeping your right heel on the floor with your toes pointing to the sky, bend your left leg and stick your backside out as you bend to create a pull on your right hamstrings. If you don't feel a pull or would like to deepen the stretch, flex the foot of the front leg so your toes point further to the sky. You can try bending the standing leg more too.

3 Stay in this position for 10 seconds.

4 Return to your normal standing position and repeat on the other side.

5 Repeat another 2 times on each leg.

You've worked on the backs of your legs; now here's an exercise for the front of your legs.

QUAD STRETCH

Stretches: quads

1 From standing still, feet hip-width apart, bend your right leg back and grab hold of your foot with your right hand. Make sure your left leg is planted firmly on the ground and that your knee is not locked. To help you stay balanced, stand facing a wall or behind a chair and hold onto it for support.

2 Your hips should be straight and your bent knee should be pointing straight down to the ground.

3 Hold this position for 15 seconds then repeat on the other leg.

4 Do both sides once more.

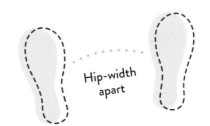

Hip-width apart

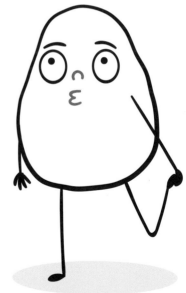

STRENGTHENING EXERCISES

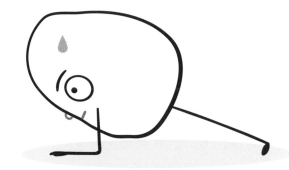

The following exercises are meant for true beginners or for those who have dabbled in exercise before but whose gym wear has not seen the light of day for many years. (The moths have probably got to them by now – it's an excuse to buy new clothes at least!) They focus on all different parts of the body with the aim of strengthening those areas. Once you've been doing the exercises regularly (that's every day) for a while, you'll notice that those body parts will start becoming more toned. That's right, defined calves can be achieved without the aid of Photoshop!

SNACK ATTACK

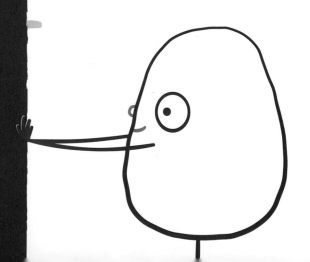

Not only a great way to fight against flabby arms, this exercise will also strengthen your willpower as you use an appliance filled with food as your gym equipment.

Tones: triceps, abs

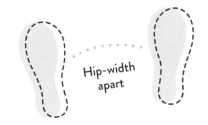

Hip-width apart

1 Position yourself next to the fridge an arm's length away and feet hip-width apart. Yep, next to the fridge – don't open it.

2 Now raise your arms to shoulder height and place on the fridge door. Start the exercise by keeping your body straight and bending your arms as you lean in towards the fridge.

3 Once your face is close to the door, push off to return to standing. Repeat this exercise until you start to tire. You'll notice that you're not only working your arms, but your stomach muscles get in on the action too.

4 You can do this against a wall but putting your weight against the fridge adds to that sense of power – you were right in front of it, but did not open it!

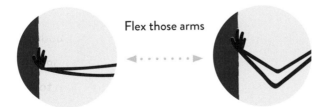

Flex those arms

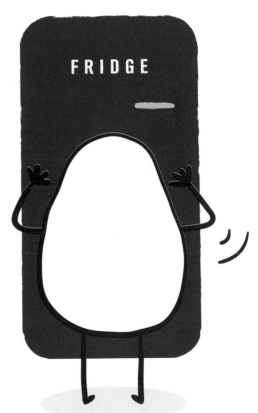

FRIDGE

LUNGE FOR FITNESS

This is a simple exercise for any place or any time you are waiting around. It can be done while making a phone call, browsing social media on your phone or waiting for the kettle to boil.

Tones: thighs and glutes

1 Stand with one leg in front of the other in an inverted "V" shape.

2 Slowly bend both your knees and lower your butt to the ground. The aim is to have both legs bent at right angles but to begin with just try to lunge as low as you can without it feeling too uncomfortable.

3 Stay at the bottom of your lunge for a couple of seconds and then slowly straighten your legs to the original standing position.

4 To begin with try
   1 lunge on each side,
and then when you feel more
confident and stronger,
increase the amount you do.

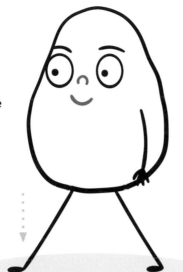

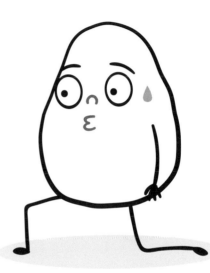

Important: when you perform a lunge make sure both feet are facing forwards. As you bend your knees, keep the front foot flat on the ground and the back heel will lift off automatically as you lower further down. Never let your front knee go over your toes – if you see this happen, it means you need to make sure your weight is in the middle of your feet, and could mean that you need to adjust your standing stance so that the "V" shape is bigger.

TURN UP THE HEAT

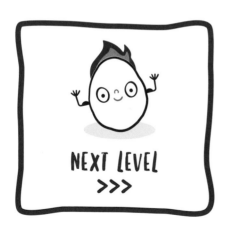

NEXT LEVEL
>>>

For something a little more challenging, try pulsing the lunges. This requires you to work on the same leg repeatedly before switching sides.

Perform your lunge and as soon as you reach your straight "V" shape, bend your knees and lower yourself back down to the bottom of the lunge again. To start with, repeat this 3 times on each leg and then swap sides. As you get fitter, increase the amount of reps you do.

There's no excuse not to perform this simple exercise as it can be done anywhere, including at home on the couch and at your work desk. You can even do it sitting on a park bench.

SIT TO GET FIT

Tones: glutes and thighs

1 So, you're in your favourite position: slouched on the couch. Drop your feet to the ground and sit on the edge of the seat.

2 Raise your arms outstretched to shoulder height keeping your feet firmly planted against the base of the couch. Now, keeping your arms stretched out in front of you, raise yourself up to standing in one fluid movement.

3 Breathe in, and sit back down again. No, don't be tempted to reach for the remote, you've got to stand up again; and repeat this exercise. Start out with 5 repetitions if you can, and build up to 10. You'll start to feel this in your thighs (your quad muscles).

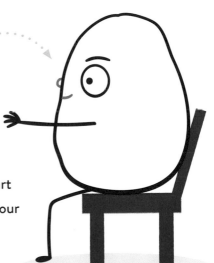

CAN LIFTS

Rummage through your kitchen cupboards for two unopened aluminium food cans. Now you're ready to work those arms!

Tones: upper arms, shoulders

1 This exercise can be done standing or sitting down. Holding a can in each hand, lift both arms so they are parallel with your shoulders.

2 Hold for 10 seconds, then lower your arms slowly.

3 Do 3 sets of 5 with 2 minutes' rest in between each set to begin with, then try to up this to 3 sets of 10.

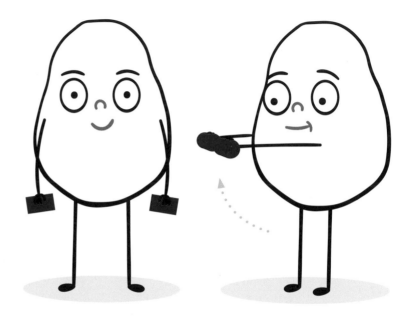

BALANCING ACT

As long as you have a steady balance this exercise is simple and the end result is beautifully shaped calves. Oh, yeah!

Tones: calves, abs

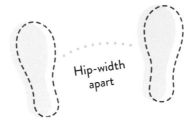

Hip-width apart

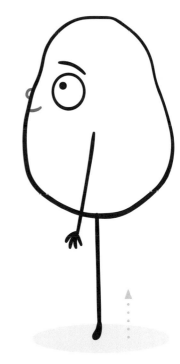

1 Stand with your feet hip-width apart and parallel. We tend to stand naturally with our weight back on our heels, so make a conscious effort to bring your weight forward slightly so your head is over your toes. Doing this and engaging your core at the same time will give you super balance.

2 Slowly rise up onto the balls of your feet – try to go through your feet so you feel all your muscles activate – and lower down in a smooth motion. If your balance is steady try to hold the position for a couple of seconds.

3 Repeat this exercise up and down on to the balls of your feet starting with 5 reps, and moving on to 10.

PILLOW KNEE-UPS

The pillow in this exercise won't be used as a comfy support for your head.

Tones: thighs and glutes

1 Hold a pillow just below shoulder height with your arms stretched out.

2 Step onto your left leg and raise your right leg high enough so it comes into contact with the pillow. If you can't lift your leg that high, lower the pillow accordingly.

3 Lower your right leg and repeat on the other side. Try to aim for 3 knee-ups on each side to begin with, and then build on this as you become fitter.

4 As you become familiar with the movement, try to speed up the sequence for a more aerobic workout.

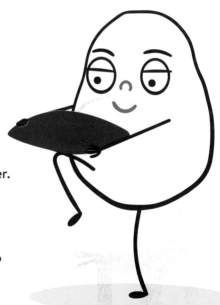

Sit and relax on a comfortable chair, and every so often raise one of your legs – it's still exercise but not the cruel type.

Tones: quads, hamstrings, abs

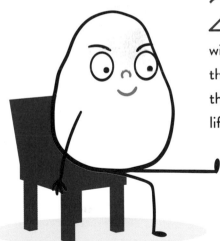

COUCH SINGLE-LEG RAISES

1 Sit with your backside perched on the edge of the couch or chair and grab the edges of the seat with your hands for extra support. Make sure your back is straight and lifted.

2 Starting with your heels touching the floor, slowly lift one of your legs in front of you as far as you can – this may be just off the floor to begin with. Grip your quad muscles to make the lift easier. The end goal is to raise them enough so they are at a right angle with your body, but this will take time. If you feel like your core can't support the lift, tilt your body back slightly.

3 Hold your leg in the air for a couple of seconds and then lower it slowly. Repeat on both legs 5 times each.

Sit on a stable chair

KNEE TO ELBOW

What better way to shape and strengthen the core than this exercise, which can be done in front of the TV while you watch your favourite programme (because who wants to miss out on a juicy plot because of exercise?!).

Tones: abs

1 Stand with your feet hip-width apart and rest your hands lightly on the back of your head.

2 Lift your left knee to waist height and twist to bring your right elbow down to meet it. Keep your back long and be careful not to hunch too much.

3 Return to the standing position and then repeat on the other side. Continue on both sides 4 more times and then have a rest. Repeat this set 4 more times.

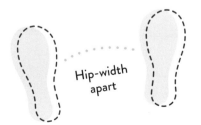

Hip-width apart

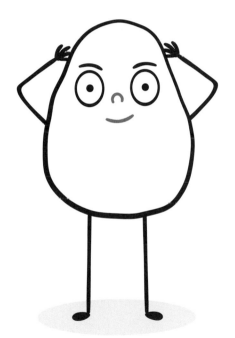

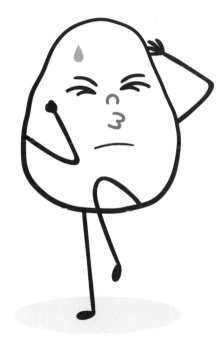

You've been practising the sit to get fit exercise (p.43), but now you think you can take it a bit further. And wouldn't it feel so amazing to be able to do a proper squat, just like the ones you see skinny minnies performing in the gym or in fitness magazines?! Hup to it then!

Tones: glutes, thighs

ALMOST-THERE SQUATS

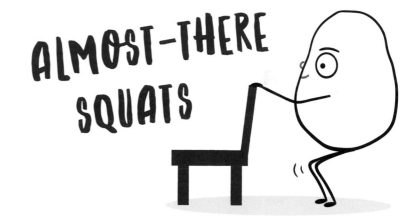

1 Standing up, place your hands on the back of a chair.

2 Position your legs so that they are about a stride away from the chair and with your feet hip-width apart.

3 Holding onto the chair, bend both knees, making sure they are parallel and not knocking into each other. Your butt should be sticking out behind you slightly. Try to lower yourself as much as you can without it feeling too uncomfortable, hold for a couple of seconds and then slowly come back up again to a normal standing position.

4 Repeat this 4 more times.

Hip-width apart

BACKWARDS LEG LIFT

When you hold this position you will feel uncannily like a dog when it goes to do its business. But don't knock it till you try it (just think of that firm butt).

Tones: glutes, thighs

1 Start by resting the weight of your body on your knees and palms, ensuring your back is straight and not bent and your hands are directly underneath your shoulders.

2 Lift one of your legs directly behind you so your thigh makes a straight line with your back and your knee is still bent at a right angle. Make sure you keep your back straight and your neck elongated (you should be looking directly down at the floor) as you raise and lower your leg.

4 Once you're used to the exercise and feel confident to build on it, you can increase the number of lifts you do or try the movement with a straight lifted leg.

3 Return to the start position and repeat the steps with the other leg. Then rest (in child pose, p.24, if you prefer).

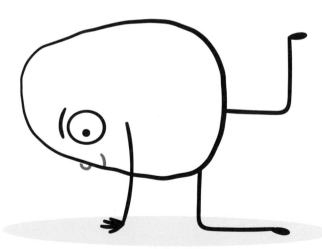

BACKWARDS ARM JAB

This may feel a little strange to your body at first – it's not a movement we perform that often, if at all – but after a while your muscles (yes, you read that correctly) will start to memorize the exercise and it will feel as normal as Friday night takeouts.

Tones: triceps

1 Kneel down on your right leg with your left foot flat out in front of you and your left knee bent upwards at a right angle. Lean your body over the left knee slightly.

2 Take your left arm and place your hand, with your fist clenched, on your left lower back, so they're gently touching. Make sure your elbow is pulled all the way back so it is facing directly behind you – if your chest

and shoulders feel open when you are doing this, you should be in the correct position.

3 Straighten your left elbow until your arm is fully stretched out behind you. (You want to try to aim for your arm to be directly behind you and not to the side. Although it will feel uncomfortable, it does provide more of a stretch and will help improve your posture.) Try to make sure your hips don't rotate as you move your arm.

4 Stay in the stretched-out position for a couple of seconds and then bend your elbow and rest your clenched fist on your lower left back again.

5 Try this movement a couple of times, then rest, then repeat on the other side. If you feel like you can do more, repeat the movement 10–15 times and then rest. Do another 2 sets of 10–15 reps, with short breaks in between, switch legs and repeat with the other arm.

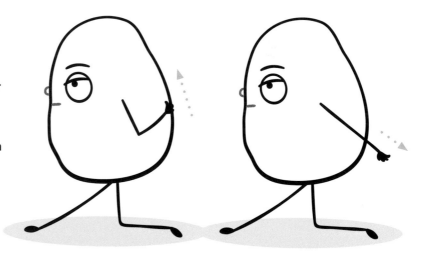

TURN UP THE HEAT

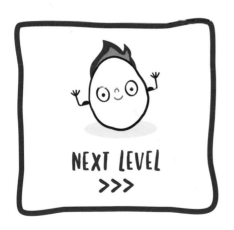

NEXT LEVEL
>>>

Do you feel like you've cracked it and want to level up? Try the backwards arm jab but hold a weight instead of clenching your fist. Use a light weight to begin with, such as a drinks can or a small bean bag, and if you feel like you could lift something a little heavier, invest in some wrist weights – they aren't expensive and can be used for many exercises in this book.

HALF PUSH-UPS

You should experiment with this exercise when you feel like the snack attack exercise (p.38) is too easy but you don't think you are ready to pull off a full push-up (p.96).

Tones: triceps, shoulders, chest and core

1 Start on your hands and knees, ensuring your back is straight and not bent, hands should be on the ground immediately beneath your shoulders. Give yourself some extra support by tucking your toes underneath your feet so they connect with the ground.

2 Imagining you are a plank of wood, keep your body rigid and bend your arms until your face is almost touching the ground and your upper and lower arms are at a right angle. Try to keep your elbows close to your body – this will make the exercise much more effective.

3 From that position, using all the arm strength you can muster, slowly push yourself back up to a flat back.

4 That's 1 half push-up complete, and may be all you can manage. If you feel like you can do a little extra, try to aim for 4 more – your arms and core might be trembling at this point, but put all your concentration into the movements and your breathing. Then have a well-deserved rest, either on your hands and knees or in child pose (see p.24). As you become stronger, you can add more to the workout.

Important: if this is your first time doing a half push-up you may want to do it in front of a full-length mirror turned on its side. This will help you to study your posture and make sure that you don't "go floppy" – a result of not using your core.

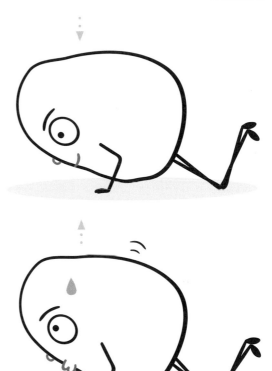

SINGLE LEG RAISES

This is a floor-based exercise to give those dormant ab muscles a wake-up call.

Tones: abs, thighs

1 Lie on your back with your arms by your sides, your knees bent and your feet flat on the floor.

2 Straighten one of your legs so that it is resting on the floor and then lift it slowly to a manageable height – make sure you engage your ab muscles at all times. Try to keep your leg lifted at the same height for 1 or 2 seconds and then lower it carefully back down to the floor, making sure it's still straight.

3   Then return to the position where both knees are bent and your feet are flat on the floor.

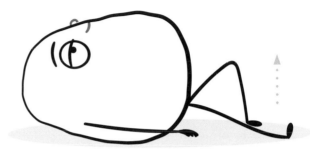

4   Rest there for a moment and then repeat with the other leg. To begin with, try repeating the exercise 5 times on each leg, and as your fitness improves you can start to add more to the sequence.

5   If you want to make it that little bit harder, perform the lift in the same way but with the non-working leg straight instead of bent.

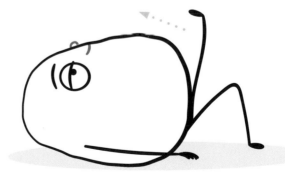

SIDEWAYS LEG LIFT

The position of this exercise may make you feel like you're in a photo shoot but it is great for the glutes and sculpting a perfectly peachy booty.

Tones: glutes, abs

1 Lie on your side with your bottom leg bent at a right angle and your top leg stretched out. Prop your head up with your hand that is nearest to the ground and place your other hand on your top hip to help stop any sideways movement when you raise your leg.

2 Slowly lift the top leg as far as it will go without your hips swaying backward or forward. Hold it in this position for a couple of seconds and then slowly lower your leg until it's resting on top of the other leg. Concentrate on isolating the movement by tensing your core so only your leg moves up and down and nothing else wiggles about. Your body should be in a straight line at all times.

3 If you feel like once is enough, rotate your body so you are lying on the other side and repeat the lift.

4 Once you start to get fitter, you can repeat the leg lift on the same side as many times as you think is enough, then have a rest. Repeat on the other side.

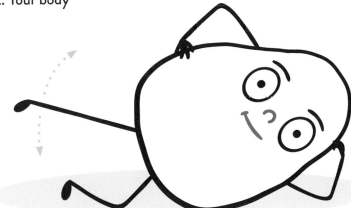

TURN UP THE HEAT

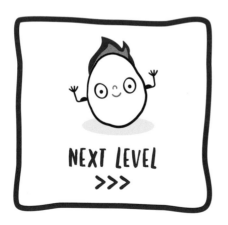

NEXT LEVEL
>>>

If you really want a hot booty (not the too-many-chillies kind though), and fast, then try this add-on for a more challenging leg lift. Lie on your side with both legs straight and wrap a resistance band around your ankles. Carry out your sideways leg lift as described on the previous page but notice how much harder it is to lift the top leg. This will give you a better butt-muscle workout.

Otherwise, try out the sideways leg lift but with an ankle weight secured to your top ankle. Or, if you are feeling brave, you could try balancing a packet of rice or pasta on your top ankle. It will probably fall off at some point but the challenge might take your mind off the exercise itself.

If at any point this feels too uncomfortable, go back to doing the basic leg lift.

BRIDGE POSE

No, we're not suggesting you go off and find a river crossing – this is another exercise that has its roots in yoga. It feels weird to begin with but after a while you'll want to do it all the time.

Tones: glutes

1 Lie down on your back and bend your knees so that you can move your feet as close to your buttocks as possible. Position your feet so they are flat on the ground and shoulder-width apart.

2 Breathe in and on the exhalation lift your backside (tense it really hard) off the floor as far as you can. The aim is for your shoulders to be the only part of your back that is touching the ground, but take it slowly to begin with and if you can only lift your buttocks off the floor, then don't attempt to go any further. Your hands should be palms down and your arms lightly touching the

floor – you don't want them to act as too much of a support otherwise you won't work your glutes properly. Whilst you are in this position scan your body and make sure that your knees are pointing directly in front of you and your chin is tucked in with your neck elongated so you can easily see your belly, and do not move your head about or twist it to the side.

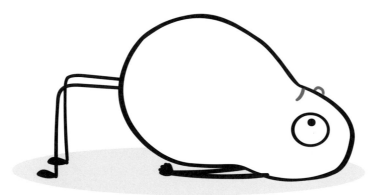

3 Hold this position for as long as you can, then carefully lower your body back to its original position with your feet still close to your backside.

4 Rest here for 20 seconds then repeat the movement as many times as you can.

TURN UP THE HEAT

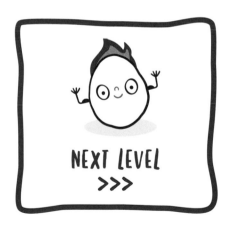

NEXT LEVEL
>>>

If you enjoy the feeling you get from bridge pose, you can feel like a true yogi by stepping it up a notch.

To open up the shoulders and chest while also working on the glutes, move your arms from by your sides to underneath you and lock your hands together by interlacing your fingers. Stay there for a few breaths then release your hands, move your arms to your side and lower yourself slowly to the ground.

BICEP CURLS

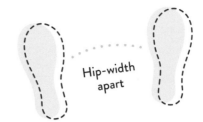

Hip-width apart

Have you ever wanted to say "Sun's out, guns out"? Yes, I thought as much! Well, soon you might be able to if you start practising this exercise.

Tones: biceps

1 Grab two small water bottles – filled not empty!

2 Stand with your feet hip-width apart and your hands by your sides with your palms facing forward, and your knees slightly bent.

3 Slowly bend your right elbow so that your right lower arm lifts all the way up till it touches your right bicep. Lower it down slowly. Make sure your back remains straight and don't be tempted to rock forwards.

4 Repeat on the other arm and then repeat an extra 9 times on both arms.

5 You can lift both weights with both arms at the same time if all you want to do is sit down and watch TV.

6 After a while you can increase the number of curls you do, taking small rests in between sets, or you can find heavier weights to do them with.

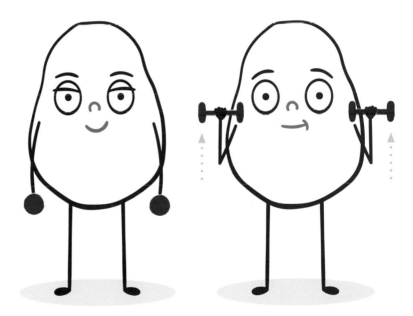

SEATED LEG LIFTS

Wow – another exercise you can do in front of the TV. This keeping fit malarkey isn't so bad after all!

Tones: abs, hamstrings

1 Sit on the floor with your legs stretched out in front of you. (Ah, so chilled.)

2 Tense your core, lean back slightly and place your hands on the ground either side of you for some extra support.

3 Slowly lift your right leg off the floor – depending on your current fitness this may be just off or at a 45-degree angle. Then lower it back to the floor slowly. Repeat with the other leg, then rest.

4 After repeating this exercise a few times on both legs you should feel a burn in your abs. (Not so chilled now.)

5 If you don't feel like your core is getting a workout, you're probably doing it wrong. The most common reason for this is that you're unknowingly tensing your quads and they are doing most of the lifting work. Always be aware of what muscles you are using and try to concentrate on your abs doing the maximum work while your legs hardly do a thing. Focusing on your breathing will help too – exhale on the lift and inhale on the release.

6 If you want to make the exercise more difficult, hold your leg at the top for longer or try to lift your leg higher. A long-term aim could be to perform 10 lifts with each leg (20 lifts in total) and then repeating this 3 times with satisfactory breaks in between.

TURN UP THE HEAT

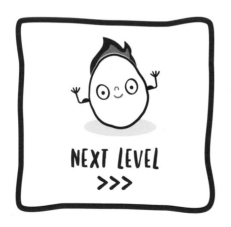

NEXT LEVEL
>>>

Don't feel like the burn is enough or maybe you enjoy the pain and want more? Whatever floats your boat, you can make this exercise more challenging by bending your knee into your chest after you've lifted it. Then straighten your leg out again, back to the position it was in, and lower it to the floor.

AEROBIC EXERCISES

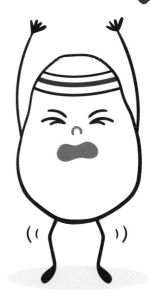

Depending on your fitness levels, you may or may not want to tackle some of these exercises. If you haven't done any exercise before or it was so long ago you can't remember, then peel your eyes away from this chapter and stick with repeating a few of the stretches and toning exercises in the previous sections. Then after a few weeks of successfully completing the exercises in those sections, you can try to combine some of the easier exercises in this chapter with the exercises you are already doing.

If you deem yourself fit enough to partake in low-level aerobic exercises such as walking at a relatively steady pace for at least 15 minutes, then you should be fine to attempt these exercises straightaway, starting with the ones at the beginning of the chapter first. However, if at any time you feel uncomfortably out of breath or experience dizziness, nausea or strain on your body and muscles, please stop whatever you are doing straightaway. If you are at all concerned with any symptoms you are having during exercising or post-workout, seek medical advice immediately.

The exercises in this chapter have been arranged in an order from easy to hard, while their introductions also give an idea of what to expect before you don your sweatbands and get into the groove. Make sure you drink plenty of water before and during exercise. Experts recommend you do 20 minutes of moderate aerobic exercises for best results, although make sure you build up to this slowly if you've never done it before.

SIDESTEP

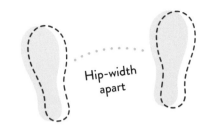

Hip-width apart

This is a gentle exercise that is great for all levels of potato (and human).

1 Stand with your feet hip-width apart.

2 Step your right foot to the side then move your left foot so it joins the right foot.

3 Repeat but step your left foot to the side and move your right foot so it joins the left foot.

4 Try doing a few of these slowly and then quicken the pace.

5 Let your arms swing naturally.

6 Continue this exercise for 2 minutes to begin with then take a rest. Then try repeating twice for another 2 minutes with breaks in between.

7   Build up the duration of the exercise as you get fitter.

8   Cool down by doing some of the stretches in the first chapter.

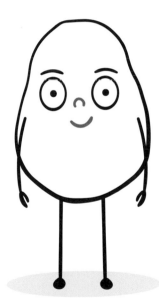
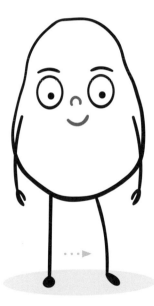
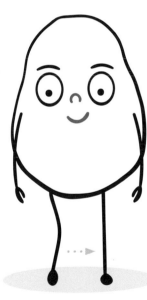

OVER THE ROPE

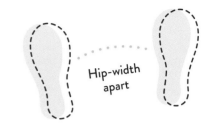

Hip-width apart

Another gentle aerobic exercise, but one that will slowly and steadily increase your heart rate.

1 For this exercise, you will need a skipping rope or anything you can find that can be laid on the floor in a straight line.

2 Place the rope in front of your feet and stand straight with feet hip-width apart.

3 Transfer your weight to your toes so your heels come slightly off the floor. This will help you to be light and springy during the exercise.

4 Take a very small jump over the rope, leading with your right foot, and follow this immediately with the left foot so that you are now in front of the rope with your weight still on the balls of your feet and your feet hip-width apart.

5 Reverse this move by springing backwards onto your right foot, followed closely by your left foot. If you don't feel confident going backwards, take the movement slowly to begin with and look back at the rope if necessary.

6 Repeat this spring forwards and backwards for 2 minutes, then have a rest. Then try repeating twice for another 2 minutes with breaks in between.

7 Build up the duration of the exercise as you get fitter.

8 Cool down by doing some of the stretches in the first chapter.

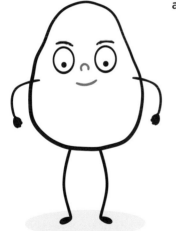

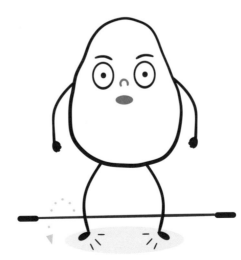

JOG ON THE SPOT

Yes, now a potato will teach a human how to run! Keep reading on to see how you can build up a sequence consisting of gentle jogging and fancy arm movements.

1 Start by jogging very gently on the spot for 30 seconds. Unlike a moving jog, you can lift up your knees slightly in front of you rather than kicking your feet behind you.

2 Now try jogging as gently as before but adding some jabs. Bend your arms into your body and clench your fists, as if shielding yourself in a boxing match. Jab your right arm in front of you until straight then bring it back close to your body and repeat with the left arm. They should be quick and fluid movements – don't forget to keep jogging!

3 Repeat this movement for 30 seconds.

4 Next, continue jogging gently with your arms bent close to your body with your fists clenched, and perform jabs like before but raise your arms so they are above your head and make a straight line vertically with your shoulders.

5 Continue this (yes, you are still jogging) for another 30 seconds.

6 Take a rest and, if you feel motivated, repeat the sequence.

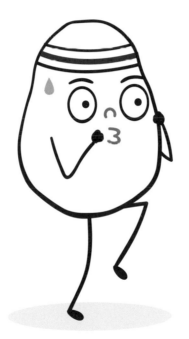

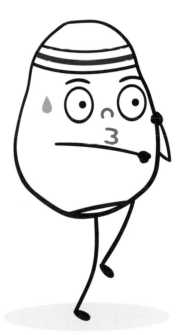

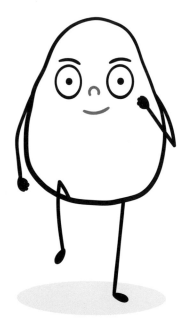

THE MARCH

You can set the tempo of this exercise to reflect your fitness levels. A good steady beat may help you to keep a regular pace. To start, you could use the music as a way to signal when to exercise and when to rest. Try completing a march to a song and when the song ends have a rest for a couple of minutes then repeat.

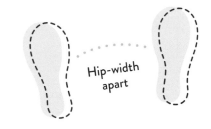

Hip-width apart

1 Begin standing with your feet hip-width apart.

2 Raise your right knee with the aim of making it parallel with your hip. If this isn't possible, just lift it as high as you can.

3 Lower your leg so your foot is flat on the ground then repeat this with the left leg.

4 Repeat this again and again, until you reach the end of the song or you feel too out of breath. A good way to tell is to try talking – if you can't this means that you should stop or slow down.

5 If you've been maintaining the same speed and you don't feel your heart rate increasing try doing the movements quicker. You could even try turning it into a knees-up jog, if you really feel motivated. Move your arms in synchronisation with your legs – keep them bent at a right angle and lift them so your upper arm is level with your shoulder.

6 Cool down by doing some of the stretches in the first chapter.

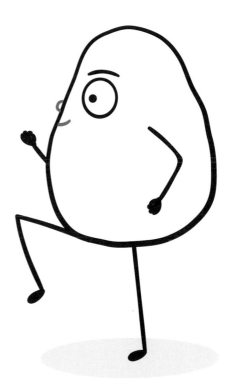

STAIR WALK

Isn't it a pain when you've just settled down in front of the TV and nature calls?! (Yes, potatoes suffer from this hindrance too!) If you start to feel like you need to go to the bathroom, use this as an excuse to perform the following exercise.

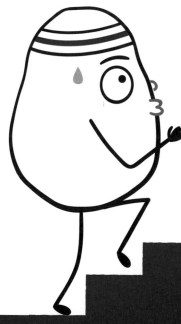

1 Walk up the stairs. (Use the facilities if bursting.)

2 Walk down the stairs.

3 Repeat.

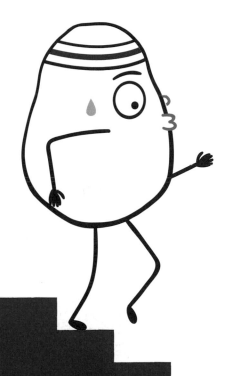

4 If you don't have stairs in your home, then today is your lucky day. (Psst – there are other exercises you can replace this with.)

5 To begin with, aim for completing 4 rounds of walking up and down the stairs. Then build on this exercise as you gain more stamina.

6 Cool down by doing some of the stretches in the first chapter.

STAR JUMPS

Hip-width apart

Jump like you mean it – this is a great exercise to do outside, either in your garden or in a park, where you can be free to stretch out as much as you like.

1 Start from a standing position, feet hip-width apart.

2 Bend your knees and bring your arms close together so your wrists are almost touching.

3 Push off your feet, jump and land your feet at the same time a little wider than shoulder-width apart. **Important:** always land your jumps with your knees bent so you don't injure yourself. As you perform this movement swing your arms out to the side and then above shoulder height so that your arms make a high "V" shape.

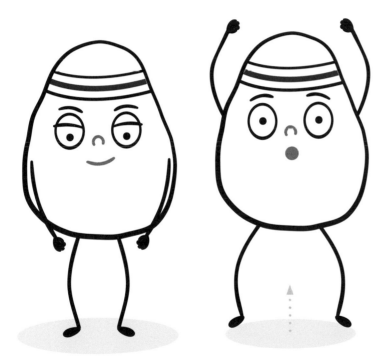

4   As soon as you reach this position, with your knees still bent, you need to push off your feet and jump them together. While you do this, swing your arms back down so they return to their original position, where your wrists are almost touching.

5   Repeat. To begin with, try performing 10 star jumps in a row. Then rest. If you felt too much strain or out of breath, don't try to do any more. If you still feel like you have some juice in the tank, try 3 sets of 10, with a break in between each set.

6   Cool down by doing some of the stretches in the first chapter.

BUTT KICKS

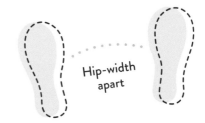

Hip-width apart

This is a compact jumping exercise that can be done in front of the TV. Prepare for your buttocks to be given a good wake-up call.

1 Start standing with your feet hip-width apart.

2 Bending your right knee, kick your right leg up behind you with enough force that your heel kicks your right glute – although not so hard that it causes pain!

3 From here, lower your leg so your right foot is flat on the ground and bring your left leg up behind you to kick your left glute. To help with balance, hold your arms out to the side at shoulder height and keep them there as you move your weight from one foot to the other.

4 Repeat this for a set of 10 then rest.

5 If you want to carry on, attempt to do 3 sets of 10.

6 Cool down by doing some of the stretches in the first chapter.

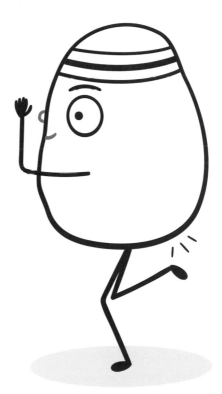

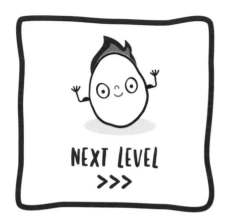

NEXT LEVEL
>>>

To make this more aerobic, try this little add-on for a harder workout.

TURN UP THE HEAT

1　Repeat the exercise on the previous page until you feel confident with the movements, but, instead of stepping from one leg to the other, try replacing the step with a little jump.

2　As you add the jump, you'll need to change your arms so that they move as they would when you jog (or see other people jog!).

3　For maximum effort, make sure you keep kicking your buttocks with your heels.

4　Try 20 butt kicks, then rest. If you feel up to it, repeat again for 2 more sets of 20.

5　Cool down by doing some of the stretches in the first chapter.

DOWN, UP, DOWN

A great exercise for all fitness needs – you'll put your lungs to the test while working on your arms and thighs without even knowing it. #likeaboss

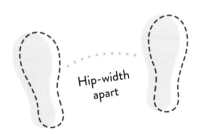

Hip-width apart

1   Start standing with your feet hip-width apart.

2   Bend your knees, curl your back and tuck your head in, so you are in a crouching position. Your heels will come slightly off the floor when you are bent all the way down. For balance, lightly rest your fingers on the floor.

3   Now here comes your extension: put your heels on the floor, straighten your knees, uncurl your back and then your head in that order. As you work through this order, slowly raise your arms so they pass along the sides of

your body, and reach up as high as you can. You can keep your feet flat on the ground or rise onto the balls of your feet, depending on how good your balance is.

4   Lower your arms and heels (if you went up on the balls of your feet) and then repeat so you lower into a crouch and then through to a big stretch standing up.

5   Repeat this 20 times and have a rest.

6   If you have the energy, continue with another 2 sets of 20 with rests in between.

7   Cool down by doing some of the stretches in the first chapter.

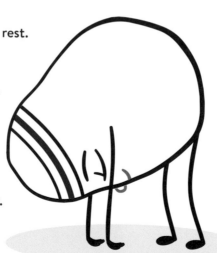

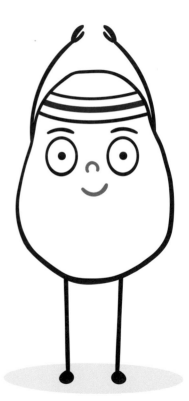

TURN UP THE HEAT

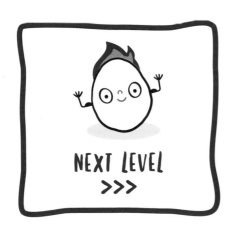

NEXT LEVEL
>>>

If you want to make this a real hot potato workout, try adding a jump into the sequence. So, from standing, you crouch down and then as you come up from standing push down on your feet and bend your knees and then jump. Go straight from the jump back down to the crouch position and repeat 20 times. Then take a rest and do another 2 sets of 20 with breaks in between.

ROCKET JUMPS

Hip-width apart

This requires a small explosion of energy – couch potatoes, are you ready for lift-off? As there's lots of vertical movement during this exercise, it's best to practise it somewhere outside unless you have high ceilings in your house.

1 Start standing with your knees bent, your feet hip-width apart and your hands resting on your thighs.

2 Push off your feet and jump as high as you can, extending your arms up straight above your head.

3 Land with bent knees – never ever try the landing with straight legs as you'll end up being a hospitalized potato – and bring your arms back down to rest on your thighs.

4 Repeat this movement another 19 times (20 in total) and rest.

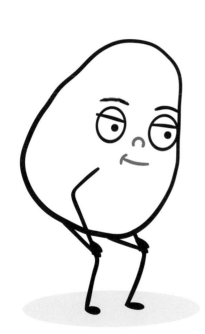

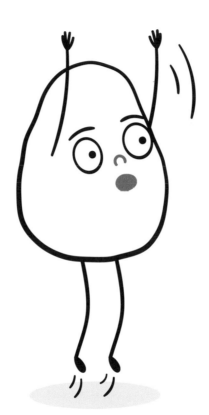

5 If you feel OK and not too exhausted, complete another 2 sets of 20 with rests in between.

6 Cool down by doing some of the stretches in the first chapter.

You've mastered the down, up, down exercise (p.87), but do you have what it takes to perform a burpee without a sit-down in between the stages? It's almost the same, just with a plank in the middle... Simple.

BURPEES

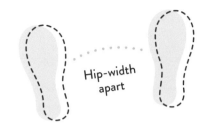

Hip-width apart

1 Start standing with your feet hip-width apart.

2 Bend your knees, curl your back and tuck your head in, so you are in a crouching position. Your heels will come slightly off the floor when you are bent all the way down. For balance, lightly rest your fingers on the floor.

3 Then move your hands so they are flat on the floor beneath your shoulders

and release your right leg behind you so it's straight and you are on the ball of your foot.

4 Then do the same with your left leg. (FYI, this is plank position – yes, you did it!)

5 Bend your right leg in, followed by your left leg so you assume the crouching position again.

6 Now here comes your extension: put your heels on the floor, straighten your knees, uncurl your back and then your head in that order. As you work through this order, slowly raise your arms so they pass along the sides of your body, and reach up as high as you can. You can keep your feet flat on the ground or rise onto the balls of your feet, depending on how good your balance is.

7 Lower your arms and heels (if you went up on the balls of your feet) and then repeat so you lower into a crouch and then through to a big stretch standing up.

8 Repeat this 5 times and have a rest.

9 If you have the energy, continue with another 2 sets of 5 with rests in between.

10 Cool down by doing some of the stretches in the first chapter.

Steps 2 and 5

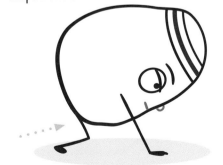

Steps 3 and 4

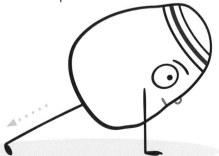

Step 7

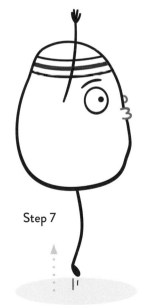

TAKING THINGS A BIT FURTHER

This chapter will look at how you can start to tone those flabby areas of your body. There's something for all parts of the anatomy, including saggy butts and upper arms. If you've been enjoying couch life a little too much over the past few years and haven't partaken in any physical exercise, this chapter isn't for you at the moment but you could definitely move onto it when your body starts to feel fitter and healthier after performing the exercises at the beginning of the book and carrying out aerobic exercise.

Note: these exercises are quite difficult so if you do fancy attempting them start by doing one practice run and then have a rest. Build yourself up slowly and if you feel like you are putting too much stress on your body, stop what you are doing immediately and once you feel better again go back to the beginners' section.

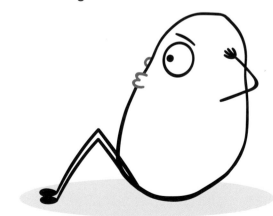

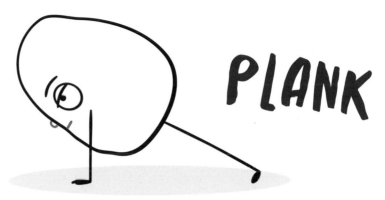

PLANK

If you are doing this position for the first time, you won't be able to hold it for long, but it is one of the best exercises for strengthening your core.

Tones: abs

1 Start by moving onto your hands and knees, ensuring your back is straight.

2 Keep your whole body stiff and rigid by gripping your abdominal muscles and shift your weight from your shins onto your toes so that your body is in a straight line on a slight diagonal (head above toes).

3 Make sure your arms are straight and your head is in line with the rest of your body. It's easy to let it hang – well, it is heavy what with all those brains – but this actually makes the exercise harder.

4 Just hold for as long as feels comfortable, then come down onto your knees and rest. Hoorah – now you can tick off planks from your exercise bucket list!

PUSH-UPS

An all-round toning triumph, this exercise requires you to assume a horizontal position but without a comfy pillow to rest your head on.

Tones: triceps, shoulders, chest and core

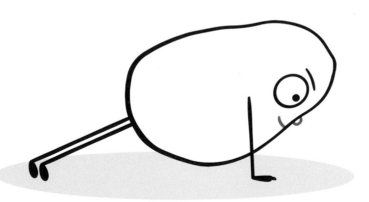

1 Start on your hands and knees, ensuring your back is straight and not bent.

2 Then prepare in plank position (p.95).

3 Imagining you are a plank of wood, keep your body rigid and bend your arms until your face is almost touching the ground and your upper and lower arms are at a right angle. Remember to always keep your elbows tucked in close to your body.

4 At this point you will be very close to touching the floor, but don't give up now and curl up into a ball – keep going! From that position, using all the arm strength you can muster, slowly push yourself back up into plank position.

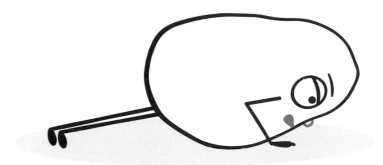

5 That's one push-up complete, and may be all you can manage. If you feel like you can do a little extra, try to aim for 4 more – your arms and core might be trembling at this point, but put all your concentration into the movements and your breathing. Then have a well-deserved rest, either on your hands and knees or in child pose (see p.24).

Important: if this is your first time doing a push-up you may want to do it in front of a full-length mirror turned on its side. This will help you to study your posture as you complete the sequence and make sure that you don't "go floppy" – a result of not using your core. Not only will going floppy make the exercise harder, but you will also struggle to lower your body without your butt staying in the air (as perfectly demonstrated by yours truly, Pot).

CHAIR-CUM-BENCH DIPS

A chair doesn't always have to be a comfortable sitting area – you can use it as apparatus for workouts too. Its multifunctional uses are perfect, as once you've completed your reps you can go back to using it as a relaxation device.

Tones: triceps

Sit on a stable chair

1 For this exercise, the chair you use needs a thin lip that is easy to grip your hands around. A desk chair without wheels is perfect – so it doesn't slide away from underneath you – but if you don't have one available, any other chair will do as long as it's sturdy, otherwise you may end up tipping it over and being stuck underneath it.

2 To get into your starting position, sit on the chair, grabbing the front of it with your hands either side of your legs, and slowly move your feet forwards so that eventually your backside slips off the chair. Once you are lifted off the chair, rearrange your position so that your knees are hip-width apart, bent at a right angle, and your back is flat.

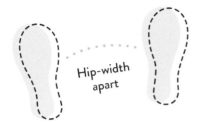

Hip-width apart

3 To complete one dip, bend your arms so that you lower your body slowly to the ground (but without sitting down, of course!). Concentrate on your elbows tucking in, as they will naturally try to open out. This makes the exercise less effective. Also check the position of your back to make sure it is still vertically straight from your head to your buttocks.

4 Hold this position for a couple of seconds, until you feel a slight burn, then come back up to the starting position. The slower and lower you dip the more effective this exercise is, but you can build up to that.

5 Try to complete 4 more in the sequence and then have a rest – on the chair if you must. As you build your strength, your aim could be to repeat the process another 4 times.

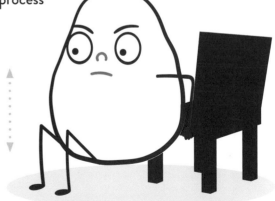

If you feel comfortable (or not too uncomfortable) doing this exercise and think you can step it up a level, try it with straight legs with your heels being your balance point and your toes pointing up to the sky. This will make it harder as your arms will be taking more of your body weight. If you are struggling,

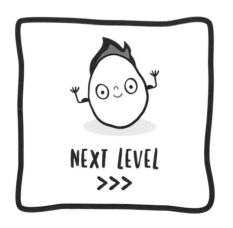

NEXT LEVEL
>>>

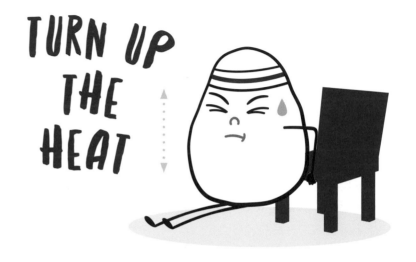

TURN UP THE HEAT

tense your core. This will help you to keep your back straight as you lower your body to the ground and will give your arms a teeny tiny bit of relief. Start off aiming for one dip to see if it feels comfortable, then gradually increase the amount you do. Always take a rest in between the dips, and if you feel yourself waning, return to doing the bent-leg version.

KERPLANK

This is tougher than your average exercise so make sure you build yourself up to it rather than making it the first you perform. The secret to introducing exercise into your everyday routine (and making it bearable) is to take small potato steps – otherwise you'll end up feeling completely mashed.

Tones: triceps, biceps, shoulders, chest and core

1 Start in the plank position (see p.95). Make sure your backside is aligned with your body and not sticking up towards the sky like a beacon.

2 Then lift off one hand and place that forearm flat on the ground. Do this with the other arm in quick succession. Your upper arms should be directly underneath your shoulders and your elbows should be bent at a right angle.

3 Hold this position for a couple of seconds and then return to the plank position with your arms stretched out. Lie

back in child pose (p.24), then if you feel like you can do more prepare in plank position again.

4 Try to do as many reps as you can without pushing yourself too hard in the first instance. You can start to build on the exercise as you begin to feel fitter and stronger.

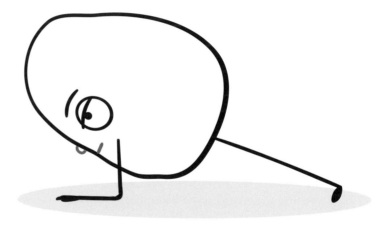

Important: the key to performing this exercise successfully is to make the movements slow and steady.

This is the go-to exercise to improve core strength and tone the abs. Some of us might know of it, but let's go back to basics and see how it's done properly.

THE SIT-UP

Tones: abs

1 Lie on your back with your knees bent up towards the sky. Keep your feet firmly on the ground at all times. (No, don't be tempted to take a nap already, we've got work to do.)

2 Engage your core and rest your hands behind your head. Slowly lift your upper back off the floor, keeping your shoulders and neck relaxed at all times. Putting strain on these muscles may cause an injury. Try not to move or tense your legs while you perform the sit-up so that the effort comes mainly from your core.

3 Doing a full sit-up on your first attempt is unheard of, so start by lifting the back of your head off the floor and then lowering it slowly and carefully, all the while relaxing your neck and shoulders and maintaining a rigid core. Repeat this a few times and then rest. Once you start to strengthen your abs, you can aim to lift your body higher. For example, the next goal might be to sit up

at just below 45 degrees, and then just above 45 degrees. Taking this exercise slow and steady is the key to strong abs without injuring yourself.

Important: don't use a prop to help anchor your feet, whether that be a small child or large adult sitting on them, or putting them underneath the couch. Having that extra support will mean that you don't need to work your abs as much and so the exercise becomes less effective. It will also start to put pressure on your lower back and could cause injury.

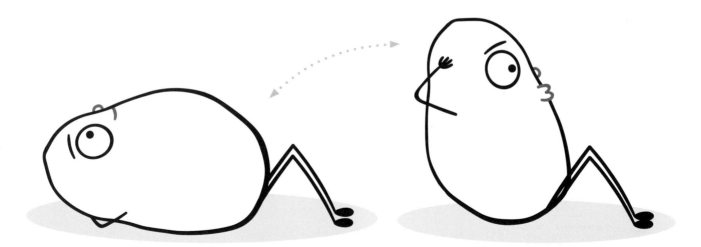

TURN UP THE HEAT

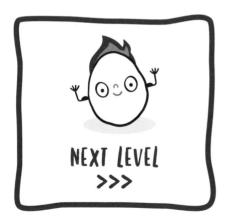

NEXT LEVEL
>>>

Once you've perfected the sit-up (or half sit-up), make your ab workouts feel more fun by turning them into a game. This is perfect if you are trying to get fit with a friend or partner. Decide how many sit-ups you want to complete, then position yourselves so that you are facing each other and a little way apart. You don't have to be able to do a full sit-up to participate – anything around the 45-degree mark is fine. Holding a small soft ball above their head, the first participant performs a sit-up. Once they reach the top of it they throw the ball to their partner who is lying down on the ground. A nice gentle throw will do so that they are able to catch it from their position. Once they've thrown the ball, the player lowers themselves carefully to the ground. Then repeat with the other player throwing the ball. Whoever drops the ball the most times has to do a set of 5 sit-ups as a forfeit (because a game without a little competition wouldn't be a game, right?!).

THE (NO-COUCH) CRUNCH

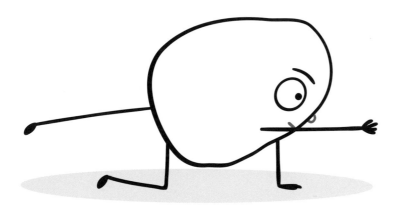

All you need is the ground beneath you for this exercise – oh, and, of course, the motivation to move onto the floor in the first place. It takes a little while to get your head around – similar to the time it takes to perfect the rubbing your stomach and patting your head conundrum – so be patient with it and take it slowly at first.

Tone: abs, glutes, shoulders, hamstrings

1 Start on your hands and knees, ensuring your back is straight and not bent.

2 Simultaneously lift your left arm out straight in front of you and your right leg out straight behind you so that your right arm and left leg are supporting your weight. Try to keep the line of your body table-top straight, including the position of your head.

3 Hold for a couple of seconds and then return your arm and leg to the ground. Repeat the movement on the other side until you become familiar with it.

4 Once you've mastered the moves, you need to add "the crunch" into the sequence. (However, if you feel that's enough for you, carry on without the crunch.) After you've performed the stretched-out position with the left arm and right leg, bring both into your body so that your elbow and knee touch. Stay here for a couple of seconds, then return to the stretched-out position and back to having both hands and knees on the floor. Again, repeat on the other side.

5 Once you feel comfortable with this, you can make the exercise more difficult by repeating the stretch and crunch multiple times without the break in between. The best way to perform exercises safely and effectively is to build on them. For example:

1 crunch on the first side, 1 crunch on the second side, rest, 2 crunches on the first side, 2 crunches on the second side, rest, 3 crunches on the first side, 3 crunches on the second side, rest, etc.

As mentioned previously, the plank is a killer exercise for firm abs. This next-level move is a great example of how you can slowly build on the basics.

Tones: abs, glutes

1 Start in the plank position (p.95).

2 Transfer your weight so that you are free to move your right leg, and bend it so it is almost touching your right elbow. Hold for a second and return to plank position or rest in child pose (p.24).

3 Then repeat on the other side. If you feel like that is enough, stop.

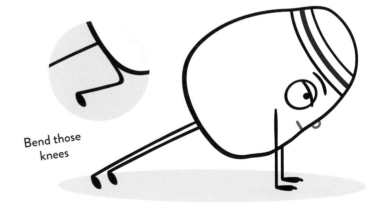

PLANK WITH LEG CRUNCHES

Bend those knees

4 As you gain fitness, you'll want to try to complete 3 sets of 5 reps and have a break in between each.

TURN UP THE HEAT

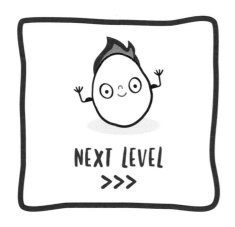

NEXT LEVEL
>>>

Getting the hang of this ab fitness stuff? Why not try an even more challenging exercise? Repeat the plank with leg crunches on the previous page but introduce an extra movement to the sequence. For example:

1 Move from plank to right leg– right elbow.

2 Then stretch your right leg back so it is parallel with your left leg but still off

the floor. This is a good point to check your posture and make sure everything is aligned properly so you are creating a nice straight slightly diagonal line from your head to your feet.

3 Continuing with the right leg, bend your knee again so your leg moves into your body but this time the aim is to make it touch or come close to your left elbow.

4 From here, stretch it out again and then lower your foot to the floor, in line with your left foot and carefully kneel down for a quick break before you repeat on the other side. For a longer rest, it can be nice to sit back in child pose (p.24).

5 This move is pretty hardcore so only attempt it if you feel confident enough.

Fancy another ab workout? Then look no further. This exercise will transform you from couch potato to smokin' hot potato.

Tones: abs

1 Lie on your back with your arms by your sides and your legs straight.

2 Keeping your legs straight and engaging your ab muscles, lift your legs simultaneously to an angle that feels uncomfortable but not painful. Then lower them (slowly if you want a stronger pull) and repeat as many times as you think is enough.

3 The aim of this exercise is to eventually raise your legs high enough so that your buttocks lift off the ground. But, hey, we can all dream right?!

DOUBLE-LEG RAISES

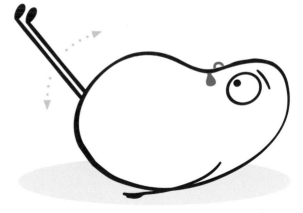

COUCH DOUBLE-LEG RAISES

You can use a couch or chair for this exercise, and you're on to a triple winner as you're toning your abs and legs simultaneously AND you can still watch TV.

Tones: quads, hamstrings, abs

1 Sit with your backside perched on the edge of the couch or chair and grab the edges of the seat with your hands for extra support. Make sure your back is straight but leaning back slightly.

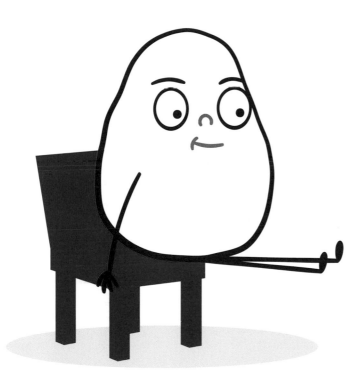

2 Starting with your heels touching the floor, slowly lift your legs as far as you can – this might be just off the floor to begin with. Grip your quad muscles to make the lift easier. If you feel like your core can't support the lift, tilt your body back even more.

3 Hold your legs in the air for a couple of seconds and then lower them slowly.

TURN UP THE HEAT

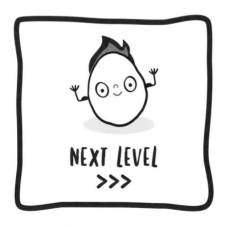

NEXT LEVEL
>>>

If you've finished your leg raises, you still have some fuel in the tank and there are 5 minutes left before your TV programme finishes, try this exercise that builds on the leg raises described on the previous page.

Repeat the lift, but once your legs are in the air, slowly draw circles with your feet. Try one rotation to begin with and then rest. If you feel up to it, try the movement again but draw 2 or 3 circles with your feet off the floor before lowering them to the ground.

To make the sequence slightly easier you can switch legs so one foot is on the ground while the other draws the circle. If you are doing it this way, try to limit movement in the resting leg to a minimum. This will make the exercise more effective.

DROP IT, SQUAT IT

The best thing about this exercise? It feels like you are just about to sit down on a chair. The worst thing about this exercise? There is no chair to sit down on.

Tones: glutes and quads

1 Stand with your feet facing forwards, hip-width apart. Put your arms out straight in front of you, palms facing the floor.

2 Perform one squat by bending your knees – visualize that invisible chair (if only it were real!). The aim is to bend low enough so that your thighs are parallel to the floor and your knees are bent at a right angle. But, for now, just try to go as low as is comfortable. Your back should be straight at all times and your knees should never be further forward than your toes.

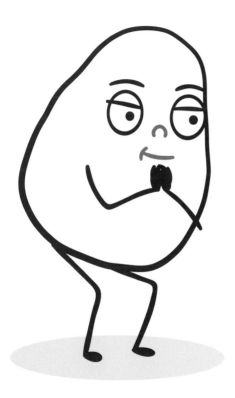

3 Sit in this position (just imagine you are chilling on a luxurious self-massage chair) for a moment if you can and then slowly straighten your knees until you are in a standing position again.

4 If you feel like that's enough, rest, but if you want to keep going aim for another 9.

5 If you don't think you can hover in this position, do the exercise with a chair/couch behind you and repeat the action of sitting and standing up (p.43).

6 Stretch out your working muscles by grabbing one foot with the same-side hand behind your body while standing straight and pull your foot towards you. You should feel a "nice" pain running through your thighs and glutes. Repeat the stretch with the other leg.

EXERCISE DIARY

To keep yourself motivated and track your progress, note down the date you exercised, what you did and what you want to achieve for next time. If you keep exercising and record your sessions consistently, you'll be amazed at what you've achieved.

Date:

What I achieved:

What I want to aim for next time:

Date:

What I achieved:

What I want to aim for next time:

Date:

What I achieved:

What I want to aim for next time:

Date:

What I achieved:

What I want to aim for next time:

Date:

What I achieved:

What I want to aim for next time:

Date:

- -

What I achieved:

- -

What I want to aim for next time:

- -

Date:

- -

What I achieved:

- -

What I want to aim for next time:

- -

Date:

- -

What I achieved:

- -

What I want to aim for next time:

- -

Date:

What I achieved:

What I want to aim for next time:

Date:

What I achieved:

What I want to aim for next time:

Date:

What I achieved:

What I want to aim for next time:

Date:

What I achieved:

What I want to aim for next time:

Date:

What I achieved:

What I want to aim for next time:

Date:

What I achieved:

What I want to aim for next time:

Date:

What I achieved:

What I want to aim for next time:

Date:

What I achieved:

What I want to aim for next time:

Date:

What I achieved:

What I want to aim for next time:

Date:
- -

What I achieved:
- -

What I want to aim for next time:
- -

Date:
- -

What I achieved:
- -

What I want to aim for next time:
- -

Date:
- -

What I achieved:
- -

What I want to aim for next time:
- -

Date:

What I achieved:

What I want to aim for next time:

Date:

What I achieved:

What I want to aim for next time:

Date:

What I achieved:

What I want to aim for next time:

Date:

What I achieved:

What I want to aim for next time:

Date:

What I achieved:

What I want to aim for next time:

Date:

What I achieved:

What I want to aim for next time:

Date:

What I achieved:

What I want to aim for next time:

Date:

What I achieved:

What I want to aim for next time:

Date:

What I achieved:

What I want to aim for next time:

THE END (BUT HOPEFULLY NOT)

You've reached the end of the book (a joyous occasion for some, I can imagine), but hopefully not the end of your path to a fitter, healthier you. This, like all good books, shows how the protagonist knew they had to change something in their life and by the end they transformed themselves for the better and discovered a more positive way to live. High-five to that! Even if you've noticed only the slightest change, this is still a massive achievement and just a glimmer of what you could accomplish. It's all about the baby potato steps! And it's not just about the difference on the scales – take note of the other changes that are happening to you, such as improved sleeping patterns and mental health, as these improvements are just as important. Keep this book on you at all times during your exercise journey to help you stay motivated and, most important of all, enjoy the ride!

Yours truly,

Instructor Pot

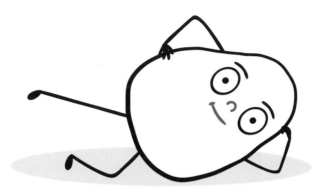

If you're interested in finding out more about our books,
find us on Facebook at **Summersdale Publishers**
and follow us on Twitter at **@Summersdale**.

www.summersdale.com

MOVEMENTS IN MODERN ART

REALISM

JAMES MALPAS

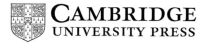
CAMBRIDGE
UNIVERSITY PRESS